Have you ever sm
that delighted yc
one that was just ...

MW01265579

Properly blending essential oils is part art and part chemistry. Just as cooking and baking utilize a recipe but generally allow some liberty with ingredients, blending essential oils will allow your creative juices to flow.

When creating blends for therapeutic effects, you may incorporate a bit of chemistry to ensure your blend does its job. But creating blends for purely aromatic purposes – to inhale, diffuse or wear as a perfume – requires more art than chemistry. With a little bit of education, a few tips and some experimentation, you will be achieving the wonderful, effective and great smelling blends you desire.

Keep in mind that this booklet contains instructions, recipes and information that should be considered a guideline for essential oil blending. There are no hard and fast rules. As with any information regarding essential oils, there will be varying viewpoints. Mine are expressed in "The Art of Blending with Essential Oils" after two decades of research and practical and clinical use. Different aromatherapy schools of thought, books and articles will only agree in part. As with most things "alternative," it is up to you, the reader, to do some research, make decisions for yourself, and use common sense when blending.

Have fun and
Get blending!

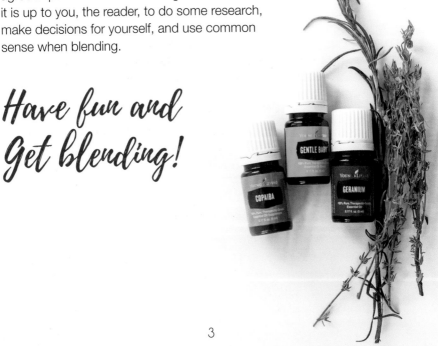

Essential Oil Basics

What are essential oils?

Essential oils are the aromatic, volatile liquids distilled from plants. Essential oils may be obtained from the seeds, roots, flowers and leaves of plants, as well as from an entire shrub or tree. Each oil may contain hundreds of molecular chemical compounds with names such as terpenes, sesquiterpenes, phenols and aldehydes, to name a few. Essential oils are very complex and currently under much study for their remarkable benefits to our wellness. For example, clary sage has 900 different molecules and lavender over 400.

How are essential oils obtained?

Steam distillation is used to release the precious oil from the majority of plants. Sophisticated and proprietary steam distillation techniques using low heat, proper pressure, precise timing, and of course fresh, properly grown and harvested plants is the only way to deliver essential oils with the quality and purity suited for blending.

Here is an example of the importance of precise timing during distillation. Properly distilled for a period of 24 hours, cypress has 280 known chemical constituents, all of which must be present for cypress to have its full complement of therapeutic benefits and potency. When distilled for 20 hours, only 20 of the 280 properties are released. If distilled for 26 hours, none of the properties are present in the resulting oil. Sadly, most cypress available in the U.S. is distilled for only about 3 1/2 hours.

Cheap, synthetic, diluted oils are potentially toxic. This is why it is so important to use only high-quality essential oils from a trusted source. The old adage "you get what you pay for" is certainly true in the essential oil industry. For these reasons, only Young Living Essential Oils are used by the author and listed in this booklet.

What are essential oil carriers?

Two types of carriers are generally used in blending. Carrier oils are fatty oils that have been pressed from a fruit, nut or seed; such as olive, sesame, coconut or almond oil. They may be used interchangeably in recipes for salves. Other carriers include water, witch hazel, and vodka, which are reserved for sprays and perfumes.

Carrier Oils

Why use a carrier oil? Many people choose to use essential oils "neat," meaning undiluted, but the real truth is that just because we CAN does not always mean this is the best method of application. Essential oil use is aromatherapy at its most potent state. Even the mildest of essential oils is very concentrated, so there are times when even one drop is more than what is needed; therefore diluting with a carrier oil becomes the best choice of application. Dilution is not just for topical use, but may also be used for inhaling, especially if you are sensitive to smells, have a lifetime exposure to home and environmental toxins, or if you are new to the world of aromatherapy. There are many carrier oils to choose from. As with all carrier oils which come from the fruit or nut of its name, these do not have the long shelf life of essential oils. Storing carrier oils in the refrigerator or a cool cabinet will help them last longer. If ever the carrier oil or blend you have made with a carrier oil smells rancid, do not use it. When possible, choose organic, less-refined carrier oils. If you purchase larger bottles of your favorite carrier oils, have a dropper bottle labeled for each, as many times the amount needed will be measured in drops, not teaspoons, tablespoons or ounces. Below are some common carrier oils and their benefits and properties:

Almond oil – from the almond nut
- Has nourishing and soothing properties for the skin.
- Suitable for babies and adults.
- Use extreme caution if you have nut allergies.

Avocado oil – from the flesh of the avocado (the part we eat)
- Very nourishing to the skin.
- Combines well with other carrier oils, due to its thicker viscosity.

Coconut oil – from the flesh of the coconut (the part we eat)
- Very nourishing to the skin.
- May cause breakouts for some people.

Grape seed oil
- Is a more astringent oil.
- Generally not used alone as the carrier oil on infants and young children, unless this astringent quality is called for.

Jojoba oil
- More of a wax than oil, though it is in a liquid state. Often used in small amounts with other carrier oils.
- Great for the scalp and softening to the skin.

Olive oil – from the fruit
- Rejuvenating and nourishing for dry skin.
- Often used in conjunction with other carrier oils because it has a stronger odor.
- When selecting olive oil, look for organic, first cold press, virgin olive oil.

Rose hip seed oil
- Should only be used in very small amounts in combination with other carrier oils.
- A very regenerative, healing oil, useful for scarring and other skin conditions.

Sesame seed oil – from the sesame seeds
- Has a very powerful odor and best left to small amounts in combinations with other carrier oils.

Sunflower seed oil – from the sunflower seed
- Has minor skin nourishing properties.
- While suitable in combination with other carrier oils, it may not be your best choice because of its strong smell.

V–6™ Vegetable Oil Complex from Young Living
- Contains the following carrier oils for the perfect blend: coconut, sesame, grape seed, sweet almond, wheat germ, sunflower, and olive.
- This is most often my first choice for blending, but, should you or a family member be allergic to one of its components, choose another carrier oil from this list.

Wheat germ oil
- Very nourishing to the skin, hair and scalp.
- Individuals who have wheat or gluten sensitivities should not use wheat germ oil.

Tips for successful blending:

- The #1 rule in blending: Keep a blending journal – Whether your blend is for aroma or therapeutic effect, you'll benefit from keeping a record of the proportions of oils used. This way you won't end up with a scent that you love but can't reproduce. If you always keep a record of all your experiments in a journal – good ones and not so good ones – once you've perfected your blend, you will be able to re-create it.

- Let it rest – It's a good idea to put a new blend away for a few days or even a week. Let the scents meld together and get comfortable with each other. Sometimes they change in ways you like. Sometimes one note becomes too strong and needs to be softened with another oil. Make a blending journal entry to adjust your blends accordingly.

- Start small – For therapeutic blends, it is smart to create a small amount and try it out to see the results. Then you can adjust your recipe until you achieve the desired effect.

Essential oil properties to remember when blending:

- Essential oils have a consistency more like water than oil, and some oils are more viscous (thick) than others. For example, vetiver is very thick, while lavender is more watery.

- Take care to avoid counteracting your formula by including two opposing singles. For example, lavender is calming while peppermint is more invigorating. Of course these two oils may be combined, but depending upon the purpose of the blend you are creating, selecting oils of the same action may be a better choice.

- Depending upon the topical application of the blend, carrier oils may be added to dilute. This can be done during the blending process or at the time of application.

- Blends may be purely essential oils, combined with a carrier oil, or in a semi-solid or solid salve or ointment.

- Roll-on dispensers for essential oil blends make for easy application. Choose cobalt blue, amber or dark green glass bottles to prevent light from damaging your blends.

- With a few exceptions, essential oils are clear in color. Some exceptions include: rose oil, which is yellowish in color; German chamomile is blue; bergamot is light to dark green; patchouli is brown or amber; and yarrow and some cypresses are blue.
- Solubility is the ability of an oil to dissolve in a liquid. Essential oils are soluble in alcohol and fixed oils, however they are not soluble in water.
- Essential oils are highly volatile, which means they readily evaporate. Each essential oil has its own volatility rate measured on a scale of 1 to 100. Essential oils with volatility rates towards 1 evaporate very quickly, whereas essential oils with volatility rates towards 100 evaporate very slowly.
- Essential oils penetrate the skin very rapidly. The time of absorption is believed to be between 20-70 minutes and varies depending upon the fat content of the skin layers of the individual.
- Some essential oils are adaptogenic, meaning the essential oil increases a person's resistance and resilience to stress, enabling the body to avoid burn out. Adaptogenic essential oils aid the body in maintaining homeostasis throughout stressful periods. Adaptogens also support the adrenal glands.
- Essential oils have minimal, if any, unwanted side effects and are known to support and enhance the body's own innate healing capacity. Essential oils are currently being explored as alternative modalities.
- When blending for therapeutic benefit, all oils combine together so long as they share the properties necessary for the conditions you are treating. Certainly some oils have a pleasant aroma when blended with certain oils, while they are less pleasing when combined with others. However, aroma should not be the primary consideration in blending unless you are simply making perfume. Choose oils based upon their therapeutic properties and focus on creating a blend based on the therapeutic benefit or purpose desired. Then you can adjust the scent when finished.

The Nose Knows

Become familiar with the scent and character of the oils. Inhale the essential oil and note how it makes you feel. Is the scent calming, uplifting, focused, sensual, happy, motivating, or energizing? Note the aroma – is it light, fresh, strong, sweet, green (like fresh mown grass), etc.?

To test the aroma of an individual essential oil, breathe directly from the bottle in the following manner: hold the bottle chest high, and gently swirl the essential oil in the bottle to stir up the molecules. Bring the bottle slowly to your nose, breathing deeply the entire time. How does it smell; how does it make you feel?

When testing several blends, you may experience olfactory overload. After a while you may no longer even be able to smell them! This is common, and you can restore your sense of smell by sniffing fresh ground coffee beans, taking a break outside in the fresh air for at least 30 minutes, or the simplest method: smell your armpit (as long as you are not wearing a synthetically or strongly fragranced deodorant). It's true – it really works and it's always with you!

Ylang ylang, myrrh or black spruce are often used as a "river" for a blend. Black spruce and rose are known to amplify the frequency of any blend to which they are added. Myrrh is known to makes a scent last longer. A river essential oil is much like a carrier oil in a blend: it acts to transport or carry the other essential oils, allowing them to blend better for fragrance purposes.

Cautions when blending essential oils:

- If you are creating a blend for someone who is pregnant, refer to *Gentle Babies: Essential Oils for Pregnancy, Childbirth and Infant Care* to wisely choose the oils.
- Clary sage should be avoided if you have endometriosis, breast, ovarian, or uterine cysts, estrogen-dependent conditions (cancers), or are pregnant.
- Avoid rosemary in excess if you have high blood pressure or epilepsy.
- Peppermint and lemon may irritate sensitive skin, so make sure they are diluted with a carrier oil or skin tested for sensitivity first.
- Bergamot, orange, lemon, and other citrus essential oils may cause sensitivity to the sun.
- Oils high in phenols and eugenol, such as oregano, thyme, clove, cinnamon, basil and tarragon, are very potent. While these powerhouses are excellent in blends, consider dilution or choosing a less-concentrated oil unless you are well-acclimated to the use of these essential oils.
- As with any new oil or blend that you use, you should check all safety data for the oils in your blend, and do a skin patch test prior to using.

So why bother to blend when there are so many existing blends for us to choose from? There are multiple reasons you might want to create your own unique blend. You may just be the creative type who wants to see what you can create. Maybe you want to turn a blend into something more like a salve. Or maybe you are in the habit of layering multiple oils and want to combine them together in one blend. And there will inevitably be a time when your favorite blend is temporarily out of stock. With a supply of many single oils, you can probably come close – or at least close enough – to creating your own substitute.

When creating blends for therapeutic benefit, the chemistry of the essential oils will be more of a factor than fragrance. However, you will want a somewhat pleasant scent to encourage regular usage. Refer to an essential oil reference book for the main chemical constituents, folklore benefits, research and properties for each single oil in your blend. The chemical constituents are often listed in order of their proportions in the oil.

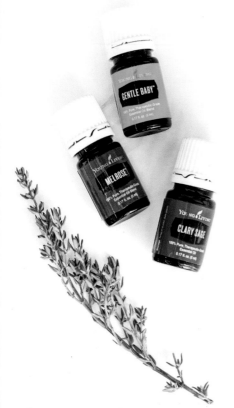

For example, if your goal is to create a blend high in monoterpenes, research the top three oils with monoterpenes and record them with their percentages in your journal. Even a blend of primarily monoterpenes, which are often soothing after strenuous work, needs more than just those compounds to make it truly effective. Sometimes it is helpful to compare your finished blend with existing blends designed for the purpose you desire.

Understanding the order in which the oils are blended is key to maintaining the desired therapeutic properties in a synergistic blend. An alteration in the sequence of adding selected oils to a blend may change the chemical properties as well as the desired results. Because your blends are for your personal use and not for resale, the order may not be such an important factor. The oils work, plain and simple. Just as when layering individual oils, the oils in a blend will absorb into the skin and do their jobs. Combining a few oils or blends into a roller ball for convenience sake will just as likely yield the same results. The order is more important, however, when a perfume or fragrance is the primary focus. For example, blends for mood support should include scents that encourage feelings of happiness and joy and will need to have a pleasing aroma, else no one will want to smell them.

Tips for therapeutic blending:

- First determine the desired effect. Choose the essential oils that may be useful – refer to aromatherapy charts that group oils according to their chemical composition in your reference books. Some suggested resources are listed at the end of this booklet.
- List essential oils in priority order when several effects are desired. This can be used to determine the number of drops of each essential oil you will use. What you want the blend to accomplish is an example of your order. However, there really is no right or wrong order in which to combine oils.
- It is important to consider all the therapeutic actions you are seeking and avoid oils that may clash with your desired goals. For instance, if you are creating a blend for muscle discomfort and sleep, peppermint and cypress can provide relief with muscle discomfort, but they are also known to promote wakefulness. You would want to avoid these oils in a blend that is intended for use right before bedtime.
- You can use approximately 5 to 28 drops of essential oil to 1/2 oz. of carrier oil, such as V-6™ Vegetable Oil Complex, in a therapeutic blend. The amount of carrier oil depends largely on the skin sensitivity of the user.

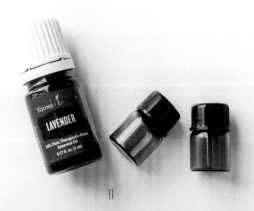

Perfume Blending

When blending for a perfume or a diffusing fragrance, the primary consideration will be aroma, and secondly, how long the scent lasts. Perfumes are a matter of personal taste: some people gravitate to fruity scents, like Young Living Citrus Fresh™, others prefer flowery scents, such as Young Living Joy™, and still others choose woody undertones, similar to Young Living Egyptian Gold™.

When creating a perfume blend, your nose may be the deciding factor, but a little instruction will help you avoid tossing a creation because of an unpleasant aroma. While there are two schools of blending, I prefer the Notes Method given below. The second method is called the Classification Method, expounded in the book *Reference Guide to Essential Oils*. (See the resources section for more information.)

While it is good to keep the following guidelines in mind for creating perfumes and diffusing blends, I have made a few great combinations by simply mixing 3-4 blends together.

> One of my most popular perfume-style blends, Momentum with Confidence, can be found in the recipe section of this booklet.

Notes Method For Creating Perfume Blends

Much like a conductor arranges his musical score based on the notes of the various instruments, essential oils have "notes" that distinguish them from other essential oils. It is these notes in the fragrance of the oil that give the plant or flower its scent. The simplest explanation of the terms top, middle and base notes is how strong and long the scent lingers. The depth, weight, or note of a specific essential oil's aroma is based on its volatility, or how fast its scent disappears or evaporates, relative to other oils. Blending a small amount of a middle note will make a top note last longer. A good way to begin blending using notes is with 30% of top note oils, 50% middle notes, and 20% base notes.

A quick way to experiment with this is to take some blotting paper, coffee filter, soft paper towels, or other absorbent paper, and drop two or three drops of different essential oils on each blotter. Try a variety of oils, such as one or two citrus oils (top notes); a woody oil like cedarwood, patchouli

A note about Notes: some oils "straddle the fence" and may fit into more than one category. This is largely due to the amount used. If you are still in doubt after trying the test above, place it in the middle.

or vetiver (base notes); and something in the middle, perhaps lavender or geranium. Set the blotters aside for a few hours before smelling them. The citrus oils are apt to have almost disappeared, while the deeper base notes should be unchanged. Check again after 24 hours, 48 hours, etc. In order for a fragrance to last a long time, a high volatility rate is preferred. If you are using an essential oil not listed below, use this evaporation method – and your nose – to find its note.

Top notes include oils such as anise, basil, bergamot, citronella, copaiba, Dorado Azul™, all varieties of eucalyptus, galbanum, grapefruit, hinoki, jade lemon, Laurus nobilis, lavender, lemon, lemongrass, lemon myrtle, orange, peppermint, petitgrain, sage, spearmint, tangerine, wintergreen and Xiang Mao.

These should make up about 30% of oils used in your blend. They are the more fruity, light, crisp scents.

Middle notes include oils such as balsam fir, black pepper, German and Roman chamomile, carrot seed, cinnamon, clary sage, coriander, cypress, dill, elemi, fennel, geranium, goldenrod, Hong Kuai, hyssop, jasmine, juniper, lavender, ledum, manuka, melaleuca, marjoram, neroli, nutmeg, ocotea, oregano, palmarosa, palo santo, pine, ravintsara, rose, rosemary, spruce, tarragon, thyme, yarrow and ylang ylang.

These should make up about 50% of oils used in your blend. These oils are the softer scents that make you say "ahhh" when you smell them.

Base notes include oils such as angelica, cardamom, cedarwood, cistus, clove, frankincense, ginger, helichrysum, jasmine, myrrh, patchouli, rose, sandalwood, vetiver, valerian and ylang ylang.

These should make up about 20% of oils used in your blend. They are the grounding, earthy, bold, rich, heavier-scented oils. Rounding the blend off with just an extra drop or so of a base note oil serves to anchor it. These oils will bring out the best in your blend and act like a river for the other oils to ride on. These base notes will often dominate a blend if you use purely equal proportions of top, middle, and base notes.

Tips for perfume blending:

- When blending perfume creations, start with small batches, using a limited amount of **4 drops of top notes, 3 drops of middle notes, and one drop of base notes**. Then you can adjust the oils to achieve the desired scent while retaining the therapeutic benefits, without using or wasting large amounts of essential oils.
- Add oils slowly, one drop at a time, to adjust the scent.
- Keep in mind that to balance the fragrance, one base note needs three middle notes and four top notes. This is a generalization, but a useful guide.

Basic Perfume Blend Recipes

Perfume with a Carrier Oil Base – for Sensitive Skin

15-25 drops of your perfume blend oils
1 tablespoon of carrier oil (V-6™ Vegetable Oil Complex, jojoba, sweet almond or apricot kernel)

Blend all oils together and store in an airtight, dark-colored glass container. Dab a drop onto your pulse points.

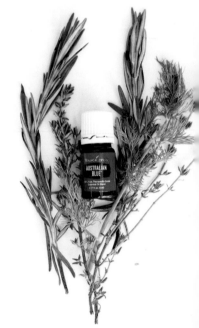

Alcohol and Water Base Perfume

4-1/4 teaspoons vodka
1-1/2 teaspoons distilled water
60 drops of your perfume blend

Combine all ingredients in a 1 oz., airtight, dark-colored glass container. Allow the mixture to sit for two weeks, swirling the bottle 1-3 times daily (more often is better) to mix the oils.

Additional procedures:

Once you have created your blend using small proportions of oils, dip a cotton swab into the blend and place it in a sealed glass container. Open and smell the mixture daily, noting any changes to the aroma in your journal. On the fourth day, check the scent, and leave the container open for 24 hours. The next day, apply a small amount to your wrists, and check the aroma immediately and once again after an hour. Note any changes to the richness or lightness of your blend to be sure you are getting the desired scent. Make adjustments by adding a drop or two of an essential oil, and start the smelling process again. Once you are satisfied with the finished product, you may make the actual amount desired. Remember, DO NOT mix more than 10-12 drops of essential oils initially because if you do not like the result, you will not have a great perfume, but an awesome-smelling toilet bowl!

Misting Blends – Perfumes and Skin Sprays

A misting blend is sprayed into the air or onto the skin. Some examples include outdoor spray, facial mist and body spray. Misting blends are typically used for their aroma, but they may also have some therapeutic benefits, such as a facial mist that nourishes the skin. A misting blend is simply a bottle with a spritzer that is filled with an appropriate blend of essential oils and water.

Misting blends must be blended in a manner that allows the essential oils to mix with the water. This is accomplished by using a blend of 50% alcohol and 50% water. Vodka is a recommended alcohol as it is relatively inexpensive and has little odor.

1. Start with 1/2 oz. of alcohol in a 1-4 oz. glass misting bottle.
2. Calculate your blend for one ounce of finished spray. Drop the essential oils in the bottle, beginning with the base notes. For a 1 oz. bottle, use approximately 20-30 drops essential oils.
3. Add 1/2 oz. of purified water and test by spraying over your head. This allows you to determine whether the scent and potency are correct. Dilute your blend by adding more water; strengthen it by adding more essential oil. Although not necessary, it may be helpful to mix the alcohol and additional drops of essential oil in a separate glass container before adding them to your blend. There is no limit to the number of drops you use in a misting blend, as they are not being applied to the body all at once. An example of a misting spray is The Great Outdoors (page 27). Notice that this blend contains 44 drops of essential oils combined with 4 ounces of water/alcohol.
4. When adjusting the scent of your spray, make sure to record each drop you add to your blend in your journal. Once you have the scent you desire, calculate the bottle size and add more alcohol, water and essential oil to reflect that multiple. Once you have determined the proportions of oils in a blend, as long as you keep the same ratio, you will produce the same scent and therapeutic value.
5. GENTLY shake your blend prior to each use.

Massage Oil Blending

A full body massage rarely incorporates more than 6-12 drops of essential oil. (Raindrop Technique is an exception.) The body should be limited to 12 drops per day when applied as a full body massage. Therefore, if you make a small blend for one massage, it should never contain more than 12 drops of essential oils, regardless of the amount of carrier oil used. Remember, a little goes a long way; oils are very concentrated. It is better to start small and add more rather than overwhelm the body.

If you are making a blend for multiple massages for one person, simply increase the number of drops used in proportion to the original recipe. Of course, the maximum number of drops per day still applies. For example, if you are making a blend intended for three massages, a maximum of 36 drops of essential oils should be used.

Please note that exceptions do apply. Use caution, and let your skin and desired results determine the amount of essential oils you use.

How to make your own salves and ointments

So why make something into an ointment or lotion? We know that oils are volatile and evaporate quickly. If you want the benefits of an essential oil to remain on your skin for a longer period of time, or if you just want a very easy method of dilution, adding essential oils to a ointment base is easy and effective.

An ointment is a preparation that is infused with herbs, essential oils for smell or added benefit, and wax to help the mixture solidify. Ointments are solid at room temperature. Salves are also infused with herbs and/or essential oils. They contain some wax to help them solidify, but they are typically more oily and loose, meaning they are less stable at room temperature. So you can see the difference is minimal. So much so that I often use the terms interchangeably, and my recipe base is the same for both salves and ointments. Commercially made products with the name balm, ointment or salve often have the same base with the primary difference being the amount of wax used to make them solid. For instance, a lip balm will contain more wax than a traditional ointment or salve.

Although salves are generally blended for therapeutic value, an appealing aroma will make the blend more pleasant to use. After you achieve your therapeutic attributes, you can adjust the blend to reflect a desired scent.

The process is simple enough, so why do some salves turn out great and others mold? And how in the world do you grate beeswax without first having a salve to treat skinned knuckles? The reason salves, creams, and ointments tend to mold is because bacteria is growing. There are a few remedies for this problem. First, check to make sure that your container is properly sterilized. If you are using herbs, keep in mind that most fresh herbs contain too much water, which will encourage mold to grow. When using fresh herbs, allow them to wilt for a few days, so that most of the moisture evaporates, before adding them to a blend. Alternatively, you can dehydrate them in a dehydrator or low-temperature oven.

For ease of use, I prefer beeswax pearls or jojoba wax beads, However, if you buy a block of beeswax instead of the little pearls, purchase a kitchen vegetable grater to be used exclusively for grating beeswax, as not all of it will wash out of the grater easily. If you spray the grater with a little vegetable oil, it will make the job much easier.

Simple Salve

Equipment needed:
Stainless steel saucepan and spoons
Fine mesh strainer or muslin (if infusing with dried herbs)
Glass measuring cup
Glass or plastic storage containers
Labels

Ingredients:
Olive oil
Beeswax
Essential oils
Dried herbs (optional)

Instructions:
Combine 1 oz. beeswax (approximately 2 tablespoons) and 1 cup of olive oil in the stainless steel pot. Heat over low heat until beeswax has melted. Allow to cool slightly before adding essential oils. Pour into your containers, let cool, label and enjoy.

Herbal Infused Salve

Ingredients:
  Cold-pressed olive oil
  Dried herbs (For 5 ounces of finished salve you need a total of 2 tablespoons dried herbs. Some options include yarrow, marshmallow, calendula flowers or rose petals.)
  Grated or pearled beeswax

1. Place herbs in a stainless steel pot with 6 oz. (2/3 cup) olive oil. Cover the pot with an oven-safe lid and place it in a 200°F oven for 2 hours. After 2 hours have lapsed, check and stir the mixture. Turn the oven off and allow the mixture to cool in the oven. The oil will be infused with all the medicinal qualities of the herbs. (Fig. 1) Alternatively, in the summer, a glass jar with the herbs and oil can be set in the sun for 6 to 8 hours.

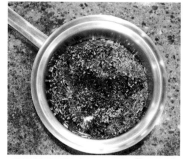

Figure 1

2. Strain the herbs through a clean piece of muslin cloth or a stainless steel fine-mesh strainer into a glass measuring cup. (Fig. 2 & 3) Allow the oil to sit for 30 minutes so that any remaining sediment can settle to the bottom. Wash out the pot, and pour the infused herbal oil back into the pot, being careful to prevent any sediment from going into your blend. You should have about 4 ounces of infused oil.

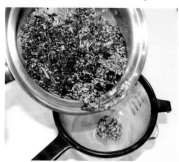

Figure 2

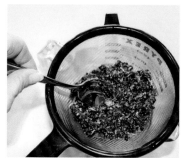

Figure 3

3. Measure 1 oz. (Approximately 2 tablespoons) of grated or pearled beeswax and add to the oil mixture. Gently warm the oil and wax mixture over medium heat until the wax melts. (Fig. 4)

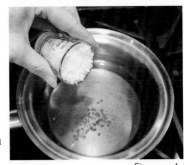

Figure 4

4. To test for correct consistency, spoon a small amount of the mixture and drizzle on a glass plate. Tilt the plate to see if the drop stays in place or runs. (Fig. 5) It should set up almost immediately. If you have to tilt it around several times before it hardens, more wax is needed. During winter months or in areas with cooler climates, salves typically set faster, and thus need less wax. If you live in warmer climates, a slightly firmer consistency will prevent your salve from softening in the heat.

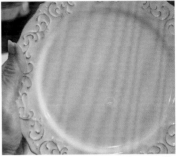

Figure 5

5. When your salve reaches the desired consistency, remove from heat and add essential oils. 40 drops of oils in a 4 oz. mixture is a good starting place. The oils will impart a therapeutic effect and also act as a natural preservative. Pour your formula into your storage containers and allow to solidify at room temperature.

   If after several hours the consistency is still too runny, scoop the mixture back into the pan, melt it, and add more wax. Heat SLOWLY and watch the mixture constantly to be sure it does not get too hot and smoke. As soon as you notice only a few bits of beeswax remaining, remove from heat and stir.

6. When solid, affix the lid and add a label. (Fig. 6) (Make sure there is no oil on the outside of the container to prevent the label from adhering. You can also place a piece of clear tape over the label to make it stay intact longer.) Be sure to keep track of your recipe and the date it was made. If it is really great you will want to make it again. Don't take chances if a formula loses its label; throw it away.

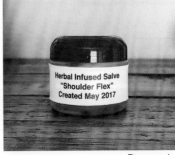

Herbal Infused Salve
"Shoulder Flex"
Created May 2017

Figure 6

Rose Ointment™ Remake Salve*

If you do not want to make your own herbal salve, salve, or ointment base, a great way to begin making creams is by using the Young Living Rose Ointment™. Rose Ointment™ is a mildly scented essential oil ointment for topical use. It is ideally suited for enhancing with more essential oils to create your personal blend.

You will need:
Young Living Rose Ointment™
Essential oils selected for your recipe – 10 drops per 2 oz. of
   Rose Ointment™
Small stainless steel saucepan (one-cup size is ideal)
Label(s) for your new creation
Optional: smaller jars for lip balms or for sharing, otherwise the new
   creation may be stored in the Rose Ointment™ jar

Visit https://vimeo.com/209236401 for a video showing this process.

1. Scoop the Rose Ointment™ into the saucepan using a small spatula.

2. Drop selected essential oils into the empty Rose Ointment™ container.

3. Warm the Rose Ointment™ on medium-high heat until melted. Remove from heat and allow to cool for 2-5 minutes. Wiggle the pan around (like stovetop popcorn) to encourage the ointment to melt at the lowest possible temperature.

4. Pour the melted Rose Ointment™ back into its container with the added essential oils. The ointment will automatically combine with the essential oils.

5. Allow the mixture to rest, uncovered, until solid. DO NOT place in the refrigerator or freezer to hasten this process, or you will be left with a "crater" in the middle of your ointment. Hardening should only take about one hour, depending upon the air temperature of your room.

6. Label your mixture appropriately, and it is ready to use.

Remember that since you are using Young Living's proprietary Rose Ointment™ as your base, you may freely use, share and give away, BUT you may not make for resale.

Blend Recipes

The following recipes will get you started using the Simple Salve, Herbal Infused Salve or the Rose Ointment™ remake salve as a base.

Notes:

- You may elect to simply create a blend of oils from the recipes below and not add them to a salve base.
- Add the following essential oil blends to one of the salve bases following the instructions above.
- When creating your own recipe, use 10 drops of essential oils per 2 oz. of ointment base. A few of the recipes below use more than this suggested amount, but these have been tested for effectiveness. As a general rule, do not use more than eight single oils or three blends in a creation. If you need more oils to get the job done, go back to the drawing board and select different oils.

Bottom's up #1 – This blend is for adults with chaffing or other minor irritation to the behind. Apply a few times daily to the area as needed.

3 drops cypress
2 drops cistus
3 drops basil
1 drop myrrh
1 drop wintergreen

Bottoms up #2 – Another variation; use as above.

4 drops cypress
2 drops myrtle
2 drops myrrh
2 drops Roman chamomile

Nail Strength, Growth & Cuticle Blend
Apply to cuticles and nails daily.

4 drops myrrh
2 drops lemon
2 drops frankincense

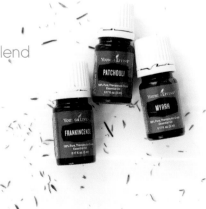

Lip Soother – Apply to chapped, dry lips.
   2 drops Melissa
   1 drop ravintsara
   1 drop thyme
   2 drops sandalwood
   2 drops lavender
   2 drops Melrose™

Female Salve #1 – This salve is great for general female chaffing, itching or redness. May be used topically or as an insertion. Caution: Do not use during pregnancy.
   1 drop clary sage
   2 drops Melrose™
   1 drop bergamot
   1 drop Melissa
   1 drop lavender
   1 drop Australian Blue™
   1 drop Roman chamomile
   2 drops mountain savory

Female Salve #2 – Similar to Female Salve #1; may be used when pregnant or nursing.
   3 drops Gentle Baby™
   3 drops 3 Wise Men™
   3 drops patchouli
   1 drop rosewood

Lip Balm – Makes eight 1/4 oz. size lip balm containers.
   3 drops myrrh
   2 drops lavender
   3 drops patchouli
   2 drops tangerine, peppermint, orange, or lemon (optional for a nice flavored lip balm)

Diaper Duty – Apply liberally to the diaper area. This works best when made into a salve.
   4 drops Gentle Baby™ or Tea Tree (*Melaleuca alternifolia*)
   2 drops lavender
   2 drops German chamomile
   1 drop cypress
   1 drop Melrose™

Wrinkles Be Gone – Add a drop to your favorite moisturizer or spot treat wrinkles you'd like to see less of.

2 drops myrrh
2 drops sandalwood
2 drops patchouli
2 drops rose
2 drops geranium
2 drops clary sage

Dry Skin

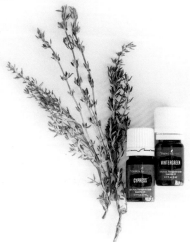

2 drops lavender
1 drop Roman chamomile
1 drop cistus
3 drops rosewood
2 drops geranium
1 drop helichrysum

BooBee Butter – Nursing Mom's Best Friend – Apply after nursing. Be sure to wipe clean before nursing to avoid an unfamiliar taste in baby's mouth.

4 drops geranium
2 drops lavender
2 drops myrrh
2 drops Gentle Baby™, Melrose™ or Tea Tree (*Melaleuca alternifolia*)

MLB – Muscles, Ligaments, Bones and Joints – Shoulders, knees, hips, backs, elbows and ankles love this blend

8 drops marjoram
8 drops lemongrass
6 drops wintergreen
9 drops PanAway™
3 drops Mister™

Skin Tightening Massage Blend – Massage a scant amount to problem areas following a shower. Another option is to combine 3 drops each of clove and copaiba with a body lotion or Cel-Light™ Magic Massage Oil, and massage into the skin.

8 drops clove
72 drops copaiba
2 ounces V6™ Vegetable Oil Complex, or carrier oil of choice

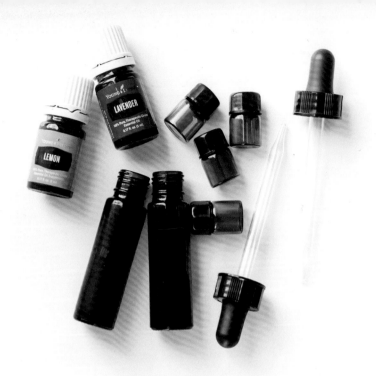

Essential oil blends not intended to be made into salves

Because of their usage, these blends are best used neat or diluted with a carrier, but not made into salves or ointments. This is my opinion; you are free to use as desired. I suggest storing in small (5 or 15 ml) bottles or roll-on bottles. You may use empty Young Living bottles, just choose a bottle that contained one of the oils in your blend, and always be sure to re-label.

Around the Eyes Blend
– Apply twice daily around the bony eye socket, taking care to not get into the eye. If you do, flush with a drop of V-6™ Vegetable Oil Complex applied to the corner of the eye. Allow it to "grab" the essential oil before dabbing with a tissue. DO NOT FLUSH WITH WATER.

   5 drops sandalwood
   5 drops juniper
   5 drops lavender
   5 drops lemongrass
   5 drops frankincense
   25 drops V-6™ Vegetable Oil Complex

Drops of Gold Facial Blend – This recipe makes 5 ounces, and is best if bottled in 1/2 oz. bottles. While this is somewhat expensive to make, you will not be disappointed with the effects of this delightful combination.

- 2 oz. almond oil
- 1 oz. jojoba oil
- 40 drops vitamin E oil
- 2 oz. evening primrose oil
- 48 drops patchouli
- 24 drops geranium
- 40 drops frankincense
- 16 drops myrrh
- 16 drops lavender
- 5 drops rose

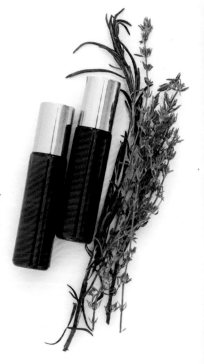

Pretty Feet Blend – Wash feet, spritz with 3% hydrogen peroxide and allow to dry. Apply 1-2 drops of this blend on and around toes and on heels.

- 5 drops oregano
- 5 drops Abundance™
- 5 drops lavender
- 5 drops thyme
- 5 drops Thieves®
- 5 drops Purification™
- 5 drops eucalyptus blue
- 1/2 oz. V-6™ Vegetable Oil Complex

Pretty Feet #2 – Clean feet well and use a bath salts recipe to exfoliate dead skin. Pat dry and apply 3-5 drops of the following blend to toes and rough heels.

- 10 drops V-6™ Vegetable Oil Complex or other carrier oil of choice
- 5 drops Tea Tree (Melaleuca alternafolia)
- 7 drops Roman chamomile
- 5 drops mountain savory
- 7 drops Laurus nobilis
- 4 drops geranium

Breast and Lymphatic Cleanse – Use neat (undiluted) on the breasts once or twice daily. A roller bottle will make for easy application.

- 5 drops Idaho balsam fir
- 5 drops ledum
- 5 drops Australian Blue™ (May substitute with 5 drops blue cypress or 5 drops cedarwood)
- 5 drops Eucalyptus radiata

Shoulder Flex – Use neat (undiluted) on the shoulders once or twice daily. A roller bottle will make for easy application.

- 5 drops Dragon Time™
- 5 drops Surrender™
- 5 drops Harmony™
- 5 drops Aroma Siez™
- 5 drops White Angelica™

Muscle Ease

- 3 drops cistus
- 3 drops marjoram
- 2 drops copaiba
- 3 drops lemongrass

Mix with 5 drops Ortho Ease® massage oil just before application, and apply at least twice per day. The use of the carrier oil is important, as lemongrass is sometimes hot to the skin.

Romantic Nights Blend – Diffuse or wear as perfume, or mist on the bed.

- 2 drops frankincense
- 1 drop ginger
- 1 drop lemon
- 1 drop orange
- 2 drops rose
- 2 drops jasmine
- 1 drop ylang ylang

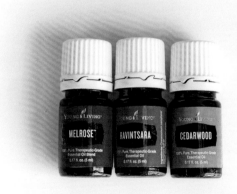

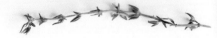

Stress Buster – For mental stress, inhale, diffuse, and/or wear this blend as perfume.

- 2 drops geranium
- 2 drops basil
- 1 drop bergamot
- 1 drop grapefruit
- 2 drops cedarwood
- 1 drop patchouli
- 2 drops Australian Blue™ (May substitute with 5 drops blue cypress or 5 drops cedarwood)

Back Rub

- 1 drop black pepper
- 2 drops helichrysum
- 1 drop marjoram
- 2 drops copaiba
- 2 drops Idaho balsam fir
- 1 drop clove

Add to 10 drops V-6™ Vegetable Oil Complex, and apply as needed.

The Great Outdoors Spray

- 10 drops lemon
- 10 drops tea tree (*Melaluca alternifolia*)
- 12 drops cedarwood
- 8 drops patchouli
- 4 drops citronella

Combine with 4 oz. water in a misting bottle, and apply outdoors.

Momentum with Confidence Perfume Spray

- 3 drops Gathering™
- 3 drops Highest Potential™
- 10 drops Sacred frankincense
- 5 drops Into The Future™
- 5 drops Motivation™
- 8 drops Believe™
- 1 drop Abundance™
- 3 drops Present Time™

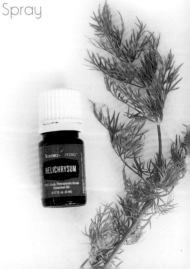

More Blend Uses

Following are some other ways to use your blends. All oil amounts are general guidelines, and you should always follow the rule that more is not always better.

Bath – Use no more than 8 drops of essential oil and even less of more potent oils. V-6™ Vegetable Oil Complex may be added to help incorporate the essential oils throughout the water. Essential oils also combine well with bath salts. Combine up to 20 drops of essential oils and one cup of bath salts (Epsom salts alone or combined with other bath salts). Use 1/4 cup per bath for a traditional sized tub; more may be used for larger tubs.

Jacuzzi – Add three drops of essential oils per person. This will evaporate almost immediately due to the heat of the water, so any benefit received is through inhalation of the essential oils. Some good choices might include mountain savory, geranium or Eucalyptus radiata.

Hot Tub Sanitizer – Use the Thieves® Household Cleaner to wipe down all surfaces before winter storage and before refilling the water. Place filters in a bucket with 15 drops Thieves® oil and enough water to cover. Soak for three hours. Replace filters, refill with water, and add 6 drops geranium oil. There is no need for harsh chemicals. (This recipe is for a 300-gallon hot tub. Adjustments can be made for a larger or smaller capacity hot tub.) *(Thanks to Richard and Shauna Dastrup, Young Living Crown Diamonds, for contributing this recipe.)*

Sauna (wet) – 2 drops per 500-600 ml water. Limit your choices to Eucalyptus radiata, *Melaleuca alternifolia* or pine, as they are excreted through perspiration after inhalation.

Diffusers – It is fun to create diffusing blends. Most diffusers will accommodate 8-20 drops of essential oil. Do not add any carrier oil to your diffuser.

Humidifiers – Add 1 to 9 drops of essential oils to your humidifier. Be aware that essential oil may damage a humidifier over time. Many families just use a cold mist diffuser instead of a humidifier.

Capsules – About 8-10 drops of oil fit in a "0" size capsule, and about 15 drops will fit in a "00" size. May cut with olive oil, if desired.

Bottling Your Creations

Why invest your time and precious oils only to bottle them in clear bottles and jars that allow light to penetrate and damage the precious blend? Essential oils should be stored in colored or opaque glass bottles. Amber is the most popular option, and blue and green are also readily available in various bottle sizes, including roll-ons. Another option is to save your empty essential oil bottles to reuse for your personal blends. Occasionally, you may wish to share a few drops of a blend with a friend, with the intent that it will be used immediately. In this case, the clear perfume sample vials are acceptable. Colored glass is more important when a blend will be stored for longer periods.

For a list of companies that sell a wide variety of glass vials, bottles and jars acceptable for essential oil creations, see the Resources section at the end of this booklet.

And remember, only the best essential oils – Young Living Therapeutic Grade essential oils – will give you the powerful results you desire. Why settle for less? Do not expect any of these formulations to give you great results if you are using anything other than pure Young Living essential oils.

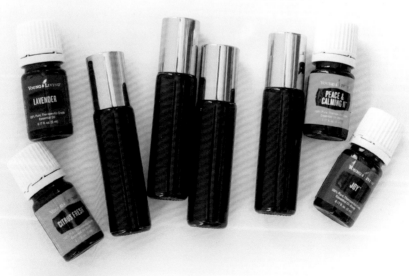

Bonus Recipe Section

Now that you're a pro, here are a few of my all-time favorite recipes for you to enjoy.

Lip Balm

> 1 oz. almond oil
> 1 oz. olive oil
> 1/4 oz. total dried herbs (try comfrey root, calendula flowers, marshmallow root, chamomile flowers)
> 1/2 oz. cocoa butter
> 3/4 to 1 oz. beeswax
> 1 tablespoon lanolin
> 1 teaspoon raw honey
> 10 drops bitter almond oil
> 5 drops desired essential oil

1. Infuse herbs in the oil and strain. (Refer to steps 1 and 2 of the Herbal Infused Salve recipe on p. 18).
2. Place infused oil in a saucepan over medium heat. Add cocoa butter, beeswax, honey and lanolin to melt.
3. Remove from heat and add bitter almond and essential oils.
4. Pour into labeled jars or tubes and refrigerate until set.

Cocoa Butter Lip Balm

> 2.5 oz. cocoa butter
> 2.6 oz. beeswax
> 1.4 oz. sweet almond oil
> Essential oils, optional

1. Place all ingredients in a stainless steel or glass saucepan and warm until everything is melted. A double boiler works best.
2. Remove from heat and add essential oils, if desired. (This recipe is fine without added essential oils. If you choose to use them, 3-5 drops are all that is needed.)
3. Once combined, pour the mixture into jars or lip balm tubes.

Note: This recipe makes 6 ounces, a lot for a lip balm, so you may divide in half; just be careful not to burn the mixture when making such a small amount. Try melting using a double boiler when cutting the recipe in half.

Jasmine Lotion

  1 teaspoon cocoa butter
  1 teaspoon beeswax
  1/4 cup apricot kernel oil
  1 teaspoon coconut oil
  1/4 cup distilled water
  1 teaspoon aloe vera gel
  1/2 teaspoon glycerin (liquid USP)
  5 drops jasmine essential oil

1. Melt the cocoa butter and beeswax over low heat, and blend in the apricot kernel and coconut oils. Allow the mixture to cool but remain a liquid.
2. In a separate bowl, combine water, aloe vera gel and glycerin.
3. Slowly drizzle the cooled oil mixture in to the bowl while beating with a whisk. Continue whisking until all oil is blended.
4. Add jasmine essential oil, and pour into a wide-mouth container.

This recipe makes about 5 ounces. This is not as firm as some lotions, but will work well in a pump container. Because it contains no preservatives, it is wise to make this in small batches and store in a refrigerator.

Face Cream – This cream starts out a bit oily, but quickly penetrates, moisturizing and leaving your skin super smooth. This recipe requires a good blender. The Vitamix® works wonderfully.

  1/3 cup cocoa butter
  2/3 cup distilled water OR 2/3 cup herbal infusion (comfrey root &
    Echinacea angustifolia root are good choices)
  3/4 cup almond or apricot oil
  1 teaspoon anhydrous lanolin
  2 tablespoons liquid lecithin
  1/2 oz. beeswax
  1/3 cup fresh aloe vera gel

1. Make cocoa butter mixture:
   • Melt cocoa butter over a double boiler.
   • If you are making an herbal infusion, add herbs to the cocoa butter and refer to steps 1 and 2 of the Herbal Infused Salve recipe on p. 18. Strain and set aside. If you are not making an infusion, add distilled water to warmed cocoa butter.
2. Make oil-wax mixture:
   • In a separate pot, melt almond or apricot oil, anhydrous lanolin, liquid lecithin, and beeswax over low heat, and set aside to cool a bit.

3. Prepare the aloe vera gel.
   - Blend aloe vera gel in a blender until frothy.
4. Add herbal infusion or cocoa butter mixture to the blender with the aloe, and blend together. Turn off blender and set aside.
5. Pour cooled oil-wax mixture into a measuring cup with a spout, and add desired essential oils. I suggest no more than 20 drops.
6. Turn blender on to highest speed. SLOWLY drizzle the oil-wax mixture into the top of the blender. Watch for a change of consistency and listen for a change of sound in the blender. It will suddenly thicken and you will hear a "glug". When this change occurs, immediately stop adding the oil mixture, even if there is some left in the measuring cup.
7. Spoon into jars and label.

Because there are no preservatives in this recipe, it is best if kept refrigerated. Stored this way, it will last approximately 3-4 months. Use twice daily for smooth, nourished skin.

Winter Weather Hand and Body Cream – Nothing soothes dry, winter skin faster than this cream. This recipe requires a good blender. The Vitamix® works wonderfully.

1/2 cup comfrey root decoction (root tea)
1 cup olive oil
1 oz. beeswax, pellets or grated
2 tablespoons liquid lanolin
3 tablespoons liquid lecithin
10 drops distilled water
10 drops essential oil

1. Make comfrey tea with 2 tablespoons comfrey root and 3/4 cup distilled water. Strain and set aside. (Yields 1/2 cup comfrey root decoction.)
2. Heat oil, beeswax, lanolin and lecithin in the top of a double boiler. Cool to a warm temperature, and stir in 2 oz. of the comfrey tea (1/4 cup).
3. Pour into blender and whip until thick and creamy.
4. Place blender jar in the refrigerator to cool. This may take a couple of hours, but DO NOT put in freezer.
5. Once the mixture is completely cooled, add essential oils and blend again until smooth.
6. Spoon into jars, label and enjoy.

Because there are no preservatives in this recipe, it is best if kept refrigerated. Stored this way, it will last approximately 3-4 months. Use twice daily to soothe dry, chapped hands.

Care & Storage of Essential Oils

Preserving your investment of precious essential oils is important and only requires a few simple steps and a little knowledge. You may choose to purchase more than you will actually use in a month in order to be prepared with a surplus of commonly used oils. We know that some oils, such as patchouli and sandalwood, actually improve with age; while others, including citrus oils, absolutes, and very thick oils, do not fair as well. Learning the four basic categories of essential oils and how to care for them will greatly preserve their potency, longevity and your investment.

When learning about the history of essential oils, archeologists discovered several vases filled with oil in King Tut's tomb. After 3,500 years, the oils, including frankincense, were still chemically viable, even though they had partially solidified in their containers. So when people ask how long the will oils last, you can tell them – about 3,500 years or so...

The Four Categories of Essential Oils

1. Pure steam distilled single oils: This includes the largest selection of essential oils. Only one type of oil is contained in a bottle with no carrier oil or extender added. Young Living's single oils are never adulterated, extended or bottled with a carrier oil. Other companies sometimes add a carrier oil to a single oil, and still call the dilution a single. So while it may be true that only one type of essential oil is in the bottle, this is not a true single oil.

Single oil *blends* are also included in this category. These are two or more single oils in the same bottle, with no carrier oil. Most Young Living blends are combinations of single essential oils mixed together without a carrier. Others may have a carrier added to improve application or viscosity (the thickness of the oil). Blends containing a carrier, as well as diluted single oils mentioned above, fall into category #2 for care and storage.

Care & storage:
Because these oils are obtained using temperatures above 212°F, the boiling point of water, subjecting them to short periods of high heat is

not a problem. If your oils get too hot, for example in a hot car or at the beach, keep the lids closed and allow them sit at room temperature for several hours before using. Storing your essential oils at normal room temperature (below 80°F) will preserve their therapeutic qualities indefinitely.

2. A blend of pure steam distilled oils: These blends include 2 or more single oils <u>with</u> a carrier oil. It is very common to have a carrier oil added to multiple singles in a blend to prevent skin sensitivities and to make the blend flow more freely when dispensing, especially when more viscous oils are used. Because a carrier oil is added, the blend will be less stable due to the nature of the pressed seed or nut oil that serves as the carrier.

Care & storage:

Oils mixed as a blend with a carrier oil; such as olive, sesame, jojoba, or almond oil, require a little more care. Because of their natural fatty nature, the carrier oil will begin to degrade over time, even without excessive heat. Carrier oil blends should stay fresh for up to a year from purchase when they are stored at normal room temperature. If you have a surplus of carrier oil blends, it may be a good idea to use them more often or store them in the refrigerator and use within two years. Don't leave these blends in your car, and take precautions to keep them cool when they are subjected to hot temperatures. The essential oils in the blends will naturally help to prevent the oxidation of the carrier oil, but not indefinitely. Even though refrigerated storage is ideal, a cool, dark closet should allow them retain their freshness for 2-3 years. *Remember – it's not about how much you store, but how much you use.*

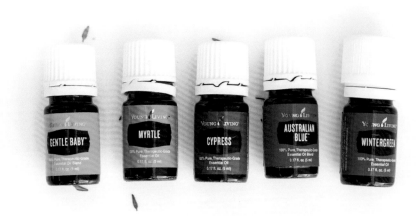

3. Cold pressed or expressed oils: This category includes oils pressed from the rind of a citrus fruit. These oils include: lemon, grapefruit, tangerine, bergamot, mandarin and lime. The rinds are pressed without heat and the oil is collected similar to olive pressing.

Care & storage:
These oils can be damaged at temperatures above 100°F and should be stored at or below room temperature. While it is fine to carry these citrus oils and blends with you, storing them in a hot car for long periods can cause their molecular structure to breakdown. Citrus oils are high in limonene, which is especially prone to oxidation. If you use your expressed oils within a year of purchase, they will serve you well, however for longer storage, refrigeration is recommended.

4. Absolutes: These oils are much more concentrated than even distilled oils. Because the delicate flowering part of the plant is used, a solvent is necessary to extract their aromatic oil. Do not let the word 'solvent' alarm you. CO_2 is the most common extraction method, and we find that used in soft drinks. While most companies use chemical solvents in which trace amounts remain in the finished product, (not only for these but also for other difficult to distill plants as well), Young Living's absolutes are processed using state-of-the-art carbon dioxide extraction technology and leaves no remaining residue.

Some plant material is too fragile to be steam distilled and this alternative method must be employed. The solvent will pull out the chlorophyll and other plant tissue, resulting in a highly colored or thick/viscous extract. The first product made via solvent extraction is known as a concrete. A concrete is the concentrated extract that contains the waxes and/or fats as well as the odoriferous material from the plant. The concrete is then mixed with alcohol, which serves to extract the aromatic principle of the material. The final product is known as an absolute. It is a very time consuming and laborious process, which is why absolutes are so costly. Examples include, but are not limited to: jasmine, rose, neroli, and onycha. These can sometimes be steam distilled, but it is more common for them to be extracted as absolutes.

Care & storage:
Absolutes can be damaged at temperatures above 90°F. Use the same care for these oils as you would for expressed oils (#3). Suggested shelf life is one year, depending upon temperature and storage conditions.

A note about oxidation: Both light and heat will eventually degrade or oxidize most oils. Although this is a slow process, it results in changing an essential oil's chemical composition and a loss of its complete therapeutic value. For this reason, essential oils should be packaged and stored in dark amber or blue glass bottles, out of direct sunlight, and in the coolest environment possible. A spare mini refrigerator is ideal but may not always be very practical. Exposure to air, such as when leaving the cap off of a bottle of oil, promotes oxidation even more than changes in temperature.

So knowing all of this you may ask, "Should I stock up?" My answer is yes. Have those oils your family uses frequently in your personal back-stock at all times. Because we must wait on plants to grow and mature before they can be harvested, the oils occasionally go out-of-stock. For this reason, I recommend keeping a 3-6 month supply. Store your stock in boxes in closed compartments of a closet, rotate them regularly, and make sure they are kept tightly capped.

Rotation is key: first in - first out.

The Bottom Line:

- Keep caps tightly closed when not in use.
- Do not store in direct sunlight.
- Avoid exposure to high heat and light for prolonged periods.
- Store at normal room temperature or cooler if possible.
- Take a periodic (now is good) inventory of your oils; rotate and use what is getting older. Use a permanent marker or colored label to denote the year purchased.
- For "sticky" oils with caps that can be hard to untwist, rub a drop of olive oil around the bottle threads, and be sure to wipe off excess essential oil after each use.
- Use your oils!

Following these simple steps will ensure your Young Living essential oils are always ready to serve you.

Essential Oil Equivalent Measurements (Approximate)

Size in ml	Number of drops	Measure	Weight/size
1 ml	15 drops	1/5 teaspoon	Fills 00 capsule
2 ml (5/8-dram bottle)	30 drops	1/2 teaspoon	1/10 oz.
3-4 ml	50 drops	3/4 teaspoon	1/8 oz.
5 ml	80 drops	1 teaspoon	1/6 oz.
15 ml	280-300 drops	1 tablespoon	1/2 oz.
30 ml	600 drops	2 tablespoons	1 oz.

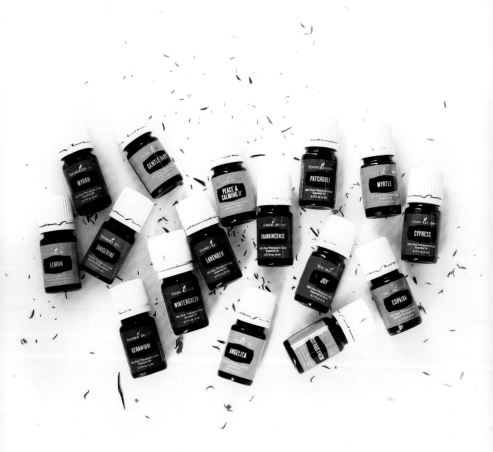

Resources

Essential Oils:
www.youngliving.com

Bottles, vials, carrier oils, beeswax and jojoba beads, dried herbs and other salve making ingredients and accessories:
www.abundanthealth4u.com
www.sks-bottle.com
www.amazon.com
www.camden-gray.com
www.etsy.com
www.herbco.com
www.starwest-botanicals.com
www.bulkherbstore.com/herbs-spices

Books:
Gentle Babies by Debra Raybern
Advanced Aromatherapy by Kurt Schnaubelt, PhD
Aromatherapy Course, Part 1, Essential Oils by Kurt Schnaubelt, PhD
Aromatherapy for Health Professionals by Shirley & Len Price
A-Z Aromatherapy by Patricia Davis
The Chemistry of Essential Oils Made Simple
   by David Stewart, Ph. D, D.N.M.
Clinical Aromatherapy by Jane Buckle, RN, PhD
Essential Oils Desk Reference Guide, Life Science Publishing
Making Aromatherapy Creams and Lotions by Donna Maria
Medical Aromatherapy by Kurt Schnaubelt, PhD
Moving Aromatherapy Forward by Kurt Schnaubelt, PhD
Natural Home Health Care Using Essential Oils by Daniel Penoel, MD
Reference Guide for Essential Oils by Connie and Alan Higley
The Complete Book of Essential Oils & Aromatherapy
   by Valerie Ann Worewood

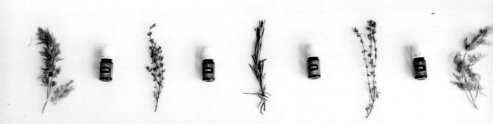